The Diabetic Diet

How to Naturally Reverse Type II Diabetes in 30 Days

Table of Contents

Disclaimer and Terms of Use:

Effort has been made to ensure that the information in this book is accurate and complete, however, the author and the publisher do not warrant the accuracy of the information, text and graphics contained within the book due to the rapidly changing nature of science, research, known and unknown facts and internet. The Author and the publisher do not hold any responsibility for errors, omissions or contrary interpretation of the subject matter herein. This book is presented solely for motivational and informational purposes only.

Introduction

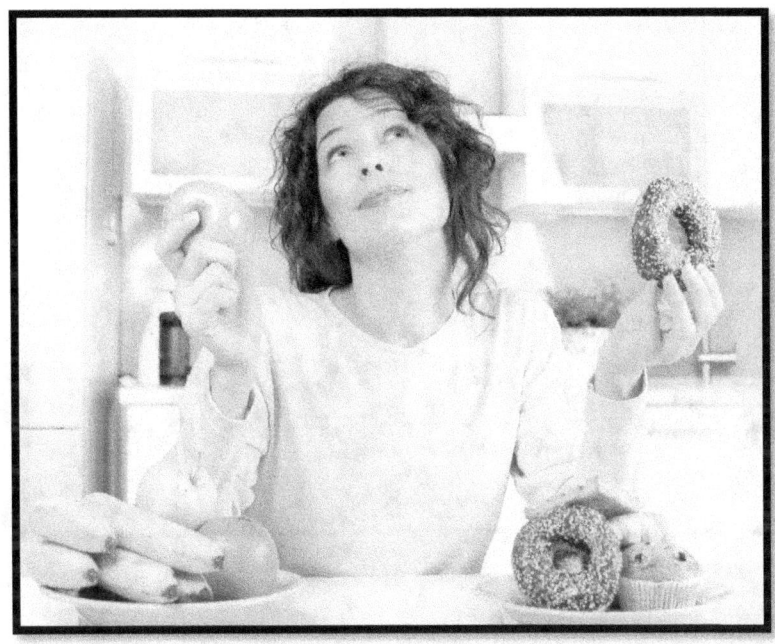

An estimated 25% of the American population is pre-diabetic and many of them do not even realize it. Diabetes is a growing epidemic in the United States, affecting over 25 million people. Each year, hundreds of billions of dollars are spent on diabetes related healthcare and the diseases causes over 70,000 deaths annually. Diabetes is the seventh leading cause of death in America and it has been linked to a number of other serious conditions including high blood pressure, kidney disease, and even Alzheimer's. If these statistics are any indication, diabetes is not a condition to be taken lightly – it is incredibly serious and, in some cases, fatal.

Whether you have been diagnosed as pre-diabetic or have already developed diabetes, do not worry – it doesn't have to be a death sentence. In fact, it is easier than you might think to control and even reverse the effects of Type II diabetes. In this book you will learn the basics about the different types of diabetes, including their causes, as well as some information about how you can reverse the condition by making simple changes to your diet. Also included in this book are tips for crafting a diabetes-reversing diet as well as recipes and a 30-day diabetes reversal meal plan. By the time you finish this book you will be equipped with the tools and knowledge to reverse your Type II diabetes or, if you are pre-diabetic, to prevent the development of the disease.

Chapter One: Understanding Diabetes

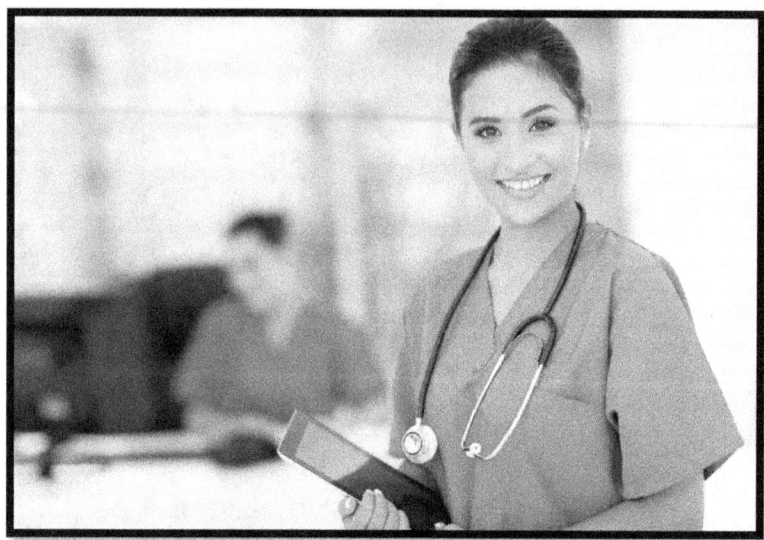

There are three main types of diabetes along with a preliminary stage referred to as pre-diabetes. Pre-diabetes is also known as glucose intolerance or impaired glucose tolerance and it is a condition in which blood sugar levels are elevated above the normal range for most people but they are not high enough to be classified as diabetic. People who have been diagnosed with pre-diabetes have an increased risk of developing Type II diabetes if they do not take steps to monitor their condition and manage their diet. The three main types of diabetes are Type I, Type II, and gestational diabetes. In this chapter you will learn about the difference between Types I and II. You will also learn about the causes for the three types of diabetes so that you may understand how making changes to your diet can help to manage or reverse your condition.

Type I vs. Type II

The main difference between Type I and Type II diabetes is that Type I is an autoimmune disease, also believed to be a genetic condition which typically presents in individuals under the age of 20. Type II diabetes, on the other hand, can develop at any age, though it is most commonly seen in adults as they get older – for this reason it is sometimes referred to as "adult onset diabetes". With Type I diabetes, the pancreas produces little to no insulin, often as a result of the pancreas being attacked by immune cells. Individuals diagnosed with Type I diabetes will require lifetime treatment with insulin shots or an insulin pump – dietary changes and health exercise habits are also recommended to help prevent extreme fluctuations in blood sugar levels.

About 90% of cases of diabetes are Type II diabetes. Whereas Type I is an autoimmune disorder, Type II diabetes is often referred to as a lifestyle disease because it is triggered by lifestyle choices an individual makes rather than genetics. Individuals who lead sedentary lives and those who are overweight are the most at-risk for developing Type II diabetes. Though this condition typically affects older adults, it is becoming more common in children and adolescents.

What Causes Diabetes?

As has already been mentioned, Type I diabetes is an autoimmune condition. What happens with individuals diagnosed with Type I diabetes is that the immune system identifies the beta cells of the pancreas (the cells that produce insulin) as foreign invaders and attacks them. As a result, the pancreas produces very little insulin or fails to produce any insulin at all. Without insulin, the individual's blood sugar levels can fluctuate drastically which leads to a variety of problems.

While in Type I diabetes the pancreas is unable to produce insulin, Type II diabetes is the result of insulin resistance. When you consume sugary foods and carbohydrates, your body produces insulin to help prevent spikes in blood sugar levels. In individuals with Type II diabetes, however, the body becomes resistant to that insulin and it takes more and more insulin to have the same effect. Over time, the body's insulin receptors get burned out and they are unable to prevent spikes in blood sugar levels any longer.

A third type of diabetes, gestation diabetes, is a condition that pregnant women can develop during the second trimester of pregnancy. Approximately 4% of women develop this condition and, unlike the other two forms of diabetes, it goes away after the child is born. Having gestational diabetes during pregnancy does, however, put a woman at a higher risk for developing Type II diabetes later in life.

Chapter Two: Making Dietary Changes

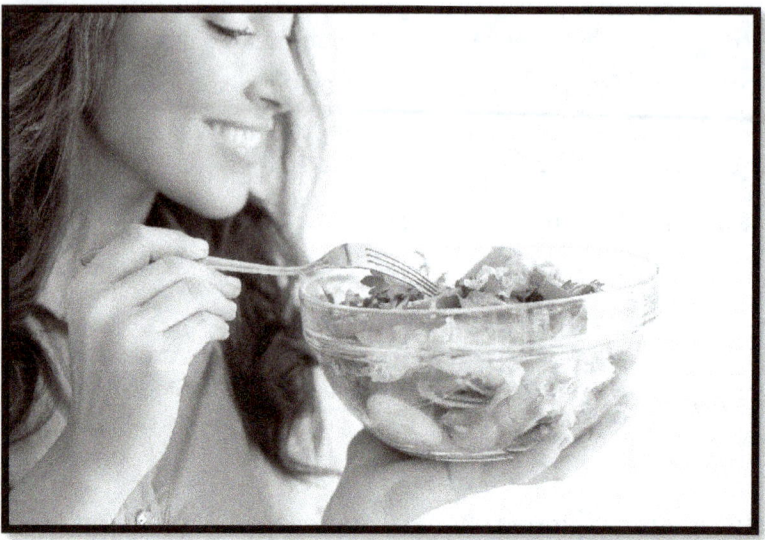

Because Type II diabetes is a "lifestyle disease," it can be reversed or "cured" by making healthy changes to your lifestyle. It is important for individuals with Type II diabetes to engage in some form of regular exercise – ideally 20 to 30 minutes of walking per day. Additionally, it is recommended that you do some form of moderate cardio or weight training 3 to 5 times per week for about 30 minutes. In addition to remaining active, there are certain modifications you should make to your diet. Certain foods that are known to cause spikes in blood sugar levels should be avoided and foods that have been shown to improve diabetes should be incorporated into your diet. In this chapter you will receive tips for removing unhealthy foods and adding healthy foods to your diet. You will also receive information about certain supplements which can help to balance your blood sugar levels.

Foods to Remove from Your Diet

The following foods have been shown to cause rapid spikes in blood sugar levels or they are, for other reasons, unhealthy for individuals with Type II diabetes:

- **Gluten-Containing Grains** – Most grains are high in carbohydrates which the body quickly breaks down into glucose. In addition to the blood sugar spiking effects of these grains on the body, gluten can also lead to inflammation which can affect your hormone levels. These, too, can lead to spikes in blood sugar levels. Refined starches and grains like white bread, white rice and white pasta are particularly damaging – whole grains are a better option.

- **Refined Sugar** – Drinking sugary beverages and consuming candy or treats can lead to sudden spikes in blood sugar levels which are very dangerous for a Type II diabetic. Glucose, the type of sugar found in these foods, is quickly metabolized by the body which means it enters the blood stream quickly. If you must use sweeteners, natural options like raw honey and maple syrup are preferable, though they should still be enjoyed in moderation.

- **Cow's Milk** – Though cow's milk is particularly problematic for Type I diabetics, it is beneficial for Type II diabetics to avoid it as well. Other forms of dairy such as goat's milk or sheep's milk are better options because they do not contain the type of A1 casein produced by commercial dairy cows that triggers an immune response in diabetics. If you do choose to consume dairy, try to stick to raw or organic products from pasture-raised animals.

- **GMO Products** – Food products like corn, soy and canola are genetically modified to enhance their growth and size. Unfortunately, these modifications change the make-up of the food which can lead to problems with the liver and kidney, particularly in diabetic individuals. It is best to remove all GMO and packaged foods from your diet as well as hydrogenated vegetable oils like canola oil and vegetable oil.

- **Alcohol** – Though there are benefits to drinking the occasional glass of red wine, most forms of alcohol are very high in sugar and carbohydrates which can lead to dangerous spikes in blood sugar levels.

Foods to Add to Your Diet

The following foods are the key to a healthy diabetes-reversing diet – add them to your daily dietary routine:

- **Whole Grains** – Though grains still contain high levels of carbohydrates, whole grains like brown rice, quinoa and whole-wheat are still better for you than refined starches. If you choose to consume grains, choose whole-grain options and limit your portions.

- **High-Fiber Foods** – Consuming high-fiber foods with each meal helps to slow your body's glucose absorption. Ideally, you should be getting at least 30 grams of dietary fiber per day from foods like nuts, seeds, vegetables, and avocados.

- **MCFAs** – Studies have shown that high intake of saturated fats can impair insulin sensitivity and that medium-chain fatty acids (or medium chain triglycerides, MCTs) are a better option. MCFAs provide the body with a quick source of fuel that is preferable to sugar (glucose) for diabetics because it does not cause a sudden spike in blood sugar levels.

- **Fish** – Wild-caught fish contain Omega-3 fatty acids which can help to alleviate some of the problems caused by elevated blood glucose levels – particularly inflammation. Studies have shown that supplementation with fish oil to increase Omega-3 levels in Type II diabetics had a positive effect on triglyceride levels without having a negative effect on glycemic control.

- **Low-Glycemic Foods** – The glycemic index is a measure of a food's ability to impact the body's blood glucose levels – high-glycemic foods have a greater effect on blood sugar levels than low-glycemic foods and are thus bad for diabetics. Some examples of low-glycemic foods that are good for diabetics to include in their diet are vegetables, nuts, seeds, avocados, coconut, eggs, wild-caught fish, pasture-raised meat, and raw dairy.

Supplements to Balance Blood Sugar

While there are no supplements out there that will "cure" your diabetes, certain supplements have been shown to help balance blood sugar levels. You may choose to take one or more of these supplements in combination with your dietary changes to help improve and reverse your diabetes. Remember, you should always check with your doctor before adding any supplements to your daily routine. The following supplements have been shown to help balance blood sugar in diabetics:

- **Fish Oil** – As was mentioned in the last section, fish oil contains omega-3 fatty acids which are necessary for proper insulin function in the body. The recommended dosage for this supplement is 1,000 mg daily.

- **Cinnamon** – You may be surprised to hear it, but cinnamon can be helpful for blood sugar control – consider adding it to your morning tea or smoothie. The recommended dosage for this supplement is 2 teaspoons daily.

- **Chromium Picolinate** – This particular supplement helps to improve insulin sensitivity in the body. The recommended dosage for this supplement is 600 mcg daily.

- **Alpha-Lipoic Acid** – This supplement helps to both reduce the symptoms of neuropathy in diabetics and improves insulin sensitivity. The recommended dosage for this supplement is between 300 and 1,200 mg daily.

- **Fiber** – As was mentioned in the last section, fiber helps to slow the body's absorption of glucose. Though eating vegetables and other high-fiber foods is good, you may want to consider a daily fiber supplement such as ground flaxseed or chia seeds. The recommended dosage for this supplement is 10 g daily.

Chapter Three: Diabetes Diet Recipes

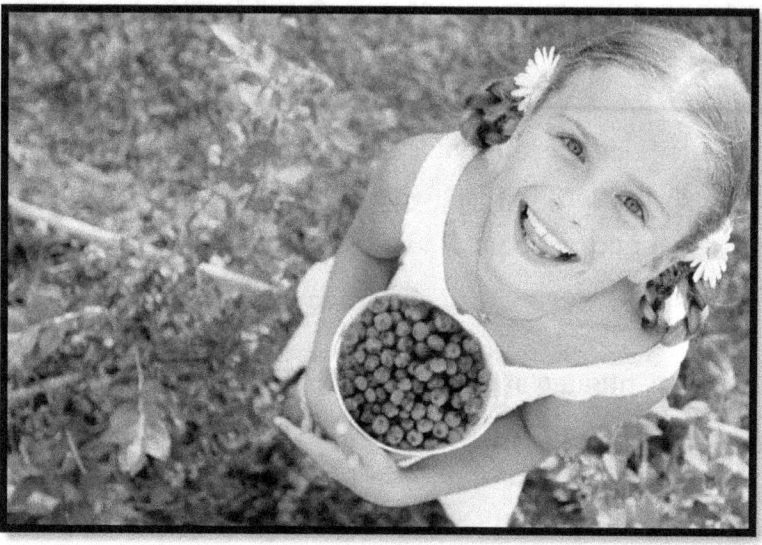

The recipes in this book are made with wholesome, natural ingredients that will help you to improve the symptoms of your Type II diabetes or to reverse it entirely. Incorporate these recipes into your daily diet along with healthy snacks. If you need help getting started with the diabetic diet, refer to the 30-day meal plan in Chapter Four.

Recipes Included in this Book:

Tropical Fruit Smoothie	Cream of Broccoli Soup	Oven-Baked Rosemary Chicken
Gluten-Free Banana Bread	Spinach Salad with Strawberries	Balsamic-Grilled Salmon Steaks
Mixed Vegetable Frittata	Corn and Black Bean Salad	Baked Halibut with Mango Salsa
Raspberry Coconut Smoothie	Coconut Vegetable Curry	Broiled Lamb Chops
Almond Flour Blueberry Muffins	Apple Pecan Chicken Salad	Asian-Style Turkey Burgers
Tomato Basil Omelet	Hearty Beef and Veggie Stew	Almond-Crusted Tilapia
Coconut Flour Banana Pancakes	Avocado Mango Spring Salad	Ginger Beef and Veggie Stir-Fry
Baked Broccoli Egg Cups	Chilled Tomato Gazpacho	Curried Lentil Stew

Tropical Fruit Smoothie

Servings: 1 to 2

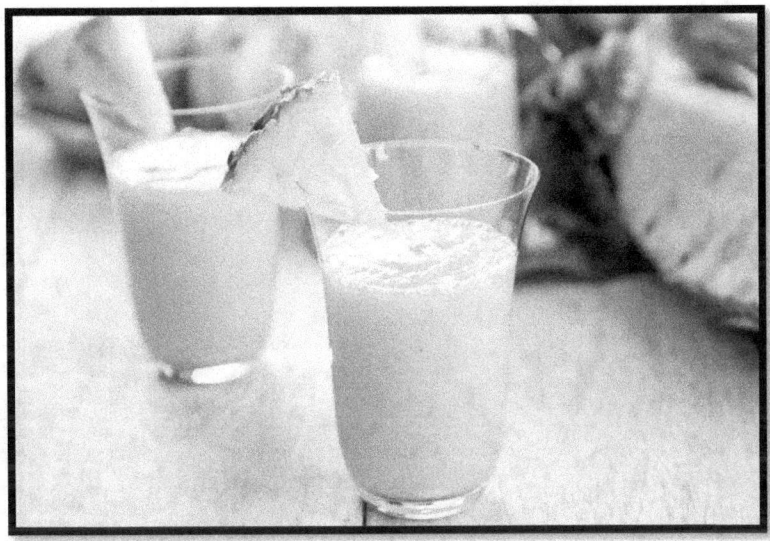

Ingredients:

- 1 cup frozen pineapple chunks
- ½ cup frozen mango chunks
- 1 ripe kiwi, peeled and sliced
- 1 cup unsweetened apple juice
- ¼ cup plain Greek yogurt

Instructions:

1. Combine the ingredients in a high-speed blender.
2. Pulse several times to chop the ingredients.
3. Blend on high speed for 30 to 60 seconds until smooth.
4. Pour into glasses and enjoy immediately.

Gluten-Free Banana Bread

Servings: 10 to 12

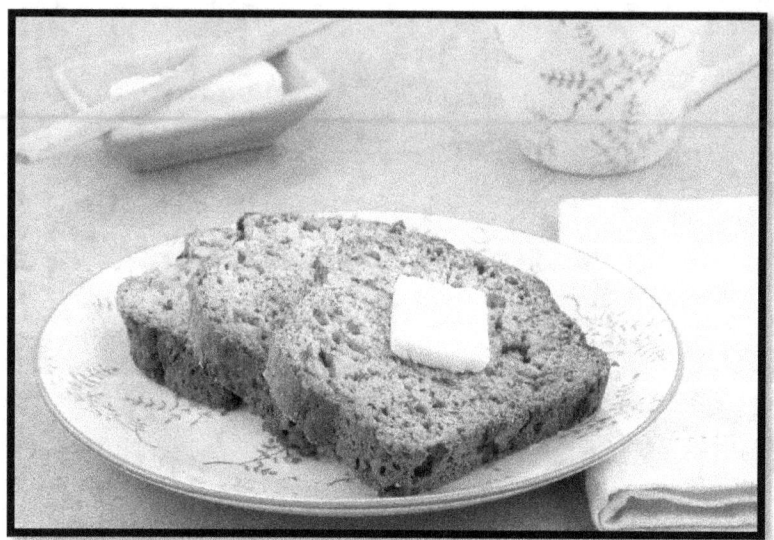

Ingredients:

- 3 medium overripe bananas, peeled and sliced
- 1 large egg, whisked
- ¼ cup coconut oil, melted
- ½ cup raw honey
- ¼ cup light brown sugar, packed
- 1 tablespoons baking powder
- 1 teaspoon ground cinnamon
- ½ teaspoon vanilla extract
- ½ teaspoon salt
- ¾ cup unsweetened almond milk
- 1 ½ cups gluten-free flour
- 1 cup almond flour
- 1 ¼ cups old-fashioned oats

Instructions:

1. Preheat the oven to 350°F and lightly grease a loaf pan.
2. Place the bananas in a large mixing bowl and mash gently with a wooden spoon.
3. Stir in the egg, coconut oil, sugars, honey, vanilla, baking powder, salt and cinnamon.

4. Whisk until well combined then whisk in the almond milk until smooth.
5. Add the remaining ingredients and stir until just combined.
6. Pour the mixture into the prepared pan and bake for 1 hour to 1 hour 15 minutes until a knife inserted in the center comes out clean.
7. Cool the loaf in the pan for 10 minutes then turn out onto a wire rack to cool completely.

Mixed Vegetable Frittata

Servings: 6

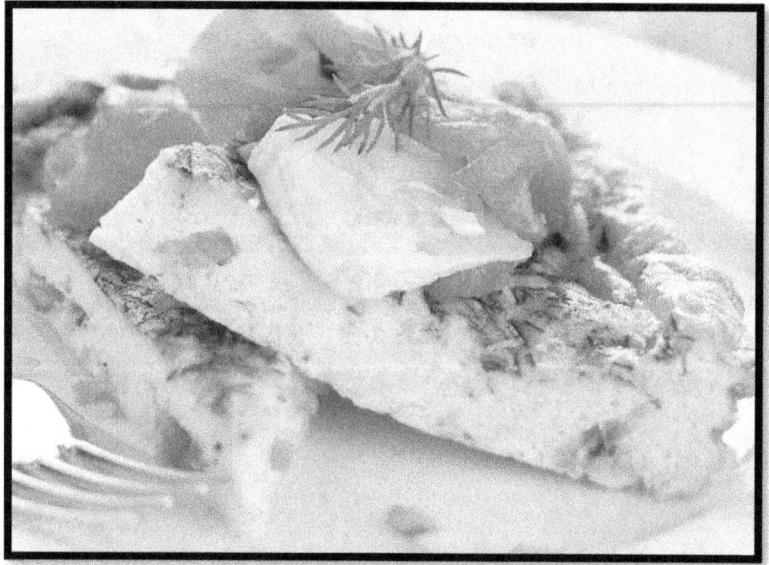

Ingredients:

- 1 tablespoon olive oil
- 1 cup diced yellow onion
- 1 teaspoon minced garlic
- 1 cup diced tomatoes
- 1 cup baby spinach, chopped
- 8 large eggs
- 2 teaspoons fresh dill
- 2 teaspoons fresh chopped basil
- Salt and pepper to taste

Instructions:

1. Preheat the oven to 375°F.
2. Heat the oil in an ovenproof skillet over medium heat.
3. Add the onion and cook for 3 to 4 minutes until translucent.
4. Stir in the garlic, tomatoes, and spinach. Cook for another 2 to 3 minutes.
5. Whisk together the eggs, dill, basil, salt and pepper in a bowl then pour into the hot skillet with the vegetables.
6. Reduce heat to medium-low and cook for 1 minute.

7. Transfer the skillet to the oven for 10 to 12 minutes until the egg is cooked through and puffed.

8. Let the frittata set for 5 minutes before serving.

Raspberry Coconut Smoothie

Servings: 1 to 2

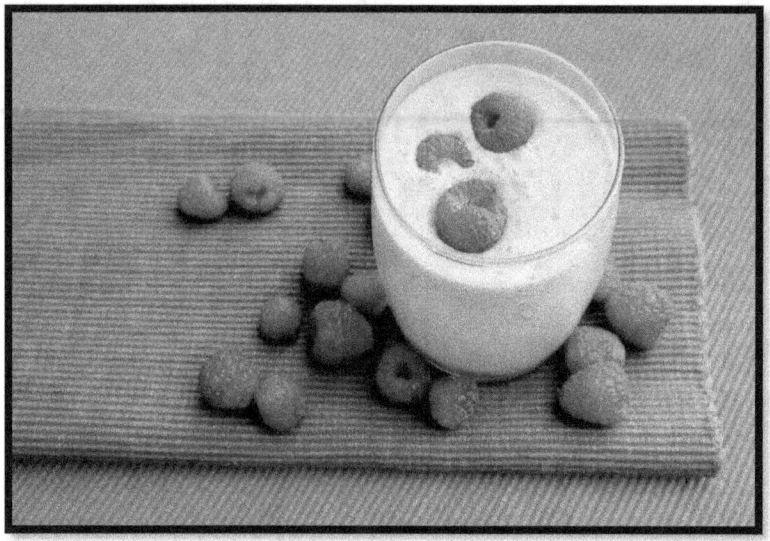

Ingredients:

- 2 cups frozen raspberries
- 1 cup unsweetened coconut milk
- ½ cup ice cubes
- 2 tablespoons shredded unsweetened coconut
- 1 teaspoon honey
- 3 drops vanilla extract

Instructions:

1. Combine the ingredients in a high-speed blender.
2. Pulse several times to chop the ingredients.
3. Blend on high speed for 30 to 60 seconds until smooth.
4. Pour into glasses and enjoy immediately.

Almond Flour Blueberry Muffins

Servings: 12

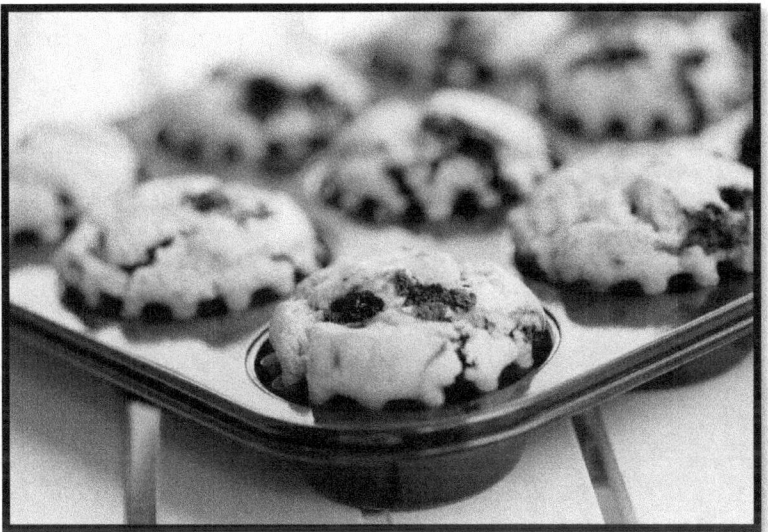

Ingredients:

- 2 ½ cups almond flour
- ¾ teaspoon baking soda
- ¼ teaspoon salt
- 3 large eggs, whisked
- ¼ cup unsweetened applesauce
- 3 tablespoons raw honey
- 2 tablespoons coconut oil, melted
- 1 teaspoon cider vinegar
- ½ teaspoon vanilla extract
- 1 cup fresh blueberries

Instructions:

1. Preheat the oven to 350°F and line a muffin pan with paper liners.
2. Stir together the almond flour, baking soda and salt in a mixing bowl.
3. In a separate bowl, beat together the eggs, applesauce, honey, coconut oil, vinegar and vanilla extract.
4. Add the wet ingredients to the dry and whisk until smooth and well combined.

5. Fold in the blueberries then spoon the batter into the prepared pan, filling the cups about 2/3 full.
6. Bake for 15 to 18 minutes until a knife inserted in the center comes out clean.
7. Cool the muffins for 10 minutes in the pan then turn out onto a wire rack to cool completely.

Tomato Basil Omelet

Servings: 1

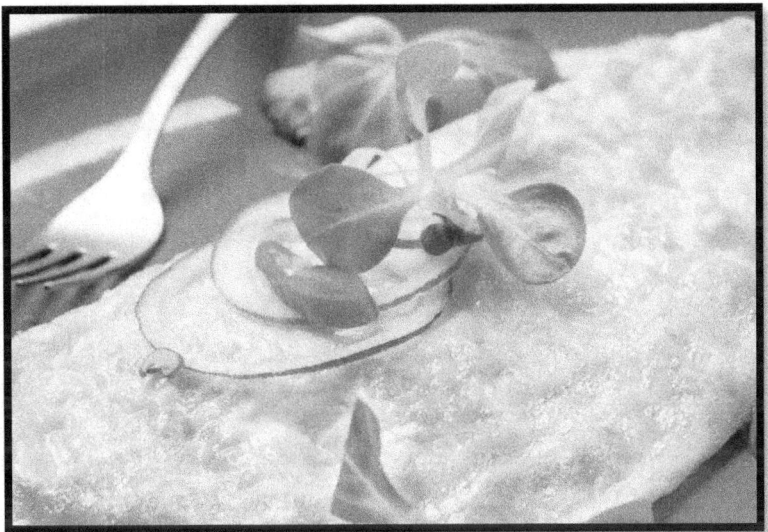

Ingredients:

- 2 teaspoons olive oil, divided
- 2 large eggs
- 1 tablespoon coconut milk
- Salt and pepper to taste
- ½ cup diced tomatoes
- 1 green onion, sliced thin
- 2 tablespoons fresh chopped basil

Instructions:

1. Heat 1 teaspoon of the oil in a small skillet over medium heat.
2. Whisk together the eggs, coconut milk, salt and pepper in a small bowl.
3. Add the tomatoes, green onion and basil to the skillet.
4. Cook for 2 minutes then spoon into a bowl.
5. Reheat the skillet with the remaining teaspoon of oil then pour in the egg mixture.
6. Cook for 2 minutes until the egg starts to set on the edges then scrape down the sides of the skillet to spread the uncooked egg.
7. Let the egg cook for another minute or two until almost set.
8. Spoon the tomato mixture over half the omelet and fold the empty half over the fillings.

9. Cook for 1 minute more until the egg is set then slide onto a plate to serve.

Coconut Flour Banana Pancakes

Servings: 4

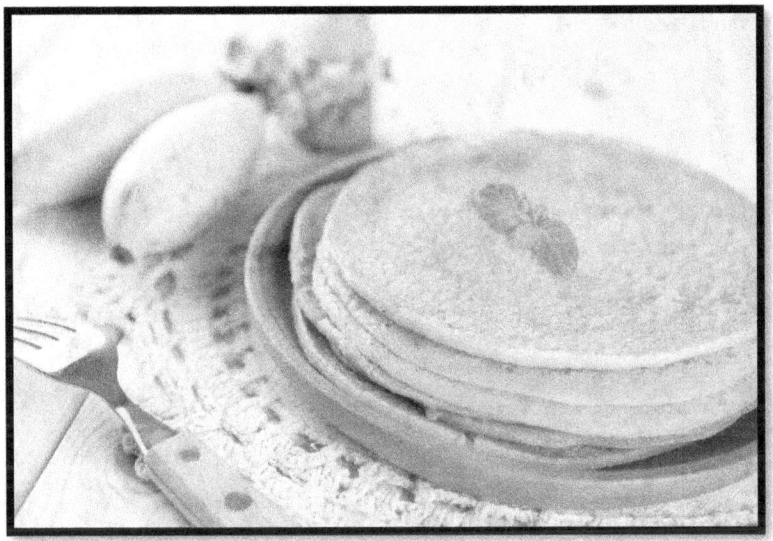

Ingredients:

- 1 cup mashed banana
- 5 large eggs, whisked
- ½ cup coconut flour
- ¼ cup coconut oil, melted
- 2 tablespoons raw honey
- 1 teaspoon baking soda
- 1 teaspoon vanilla extract
- Pinch salt

Instructions:

1. Combine all of the ingredients in a food processor and blend until smooth and well combined.
2. Grease a large skillet and heat it over medium-high heat.
3. Spoon the batter into the hot skillet using about 3 to 4 tablespoons per pancake.
4. Cook for 1 to 2 minutes until bubbles form on the surface of each pancake.
5. Carefully flip the pancakes and cook for another minute or two until lightly browned on the underside.
6. Transfer the pancakes to a plate to keep warm then repeat with the remaining batter.

Baked Broccoli Egg Cups
_____

Servings: 12

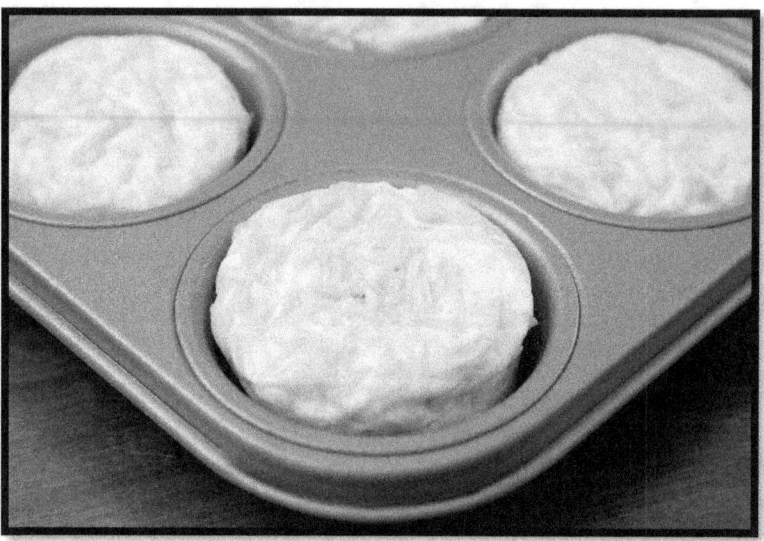

Ingredients:

- 12 large eggs, whisked
- ½ cup unsweetened almond milk
- 1 cup frozen broccoli, thawed and chopped
- ½ cup shredded cheddar cheese (optional)
- ¾ teaspoon salt
- ¼ teaspoon black pepper

Instructions:

1. Preheat the oven to 350°F and lightly grease a regular muffin pan with cooking spray.
2. Whisk together all the ingredients in a mixing bowl.
3. Pour the mixture into the muffin pan, filling the cups almost completely full.
4. Bake for 18 to 20 minutes until the egg is set in the center.
5. Cool the egg cups for 2 to 3 minutes before serving.

Cream of Broccoli Soup

Servings: 4

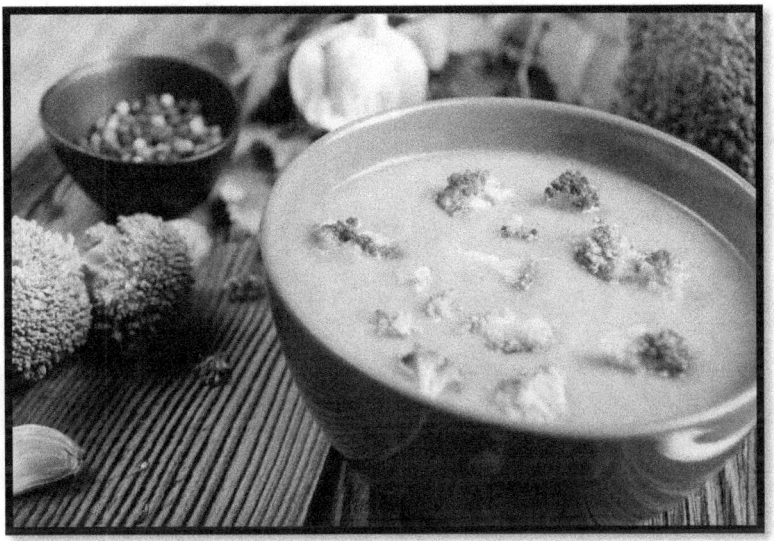

Ingredients:

- 1 ¼ lbs. fresh broccoli florets, chopped
- 2 cups vegetable broth
- 1 cup canned coconut milk
- 2 ½ tablespoons coconut oil
- Salt and pepper to taste

Instructions:

1. Bring a large pot of salted water to boil and add the broccoli.
2. Cook the broccoli for about 5 minutes until bright green and tender. Drain and set aside.
3. Whisk together the broth and coconut milk in a large saucepan.
4. Bring the mixture to a boil then add the broccoli and coconut oil.
5. Stir well and season with salt and pepper to taste.
6. Remove from heat and puree the soup using an immersion blender. Serve hot.

Spinach Salad with Strawberries

Servings: 4

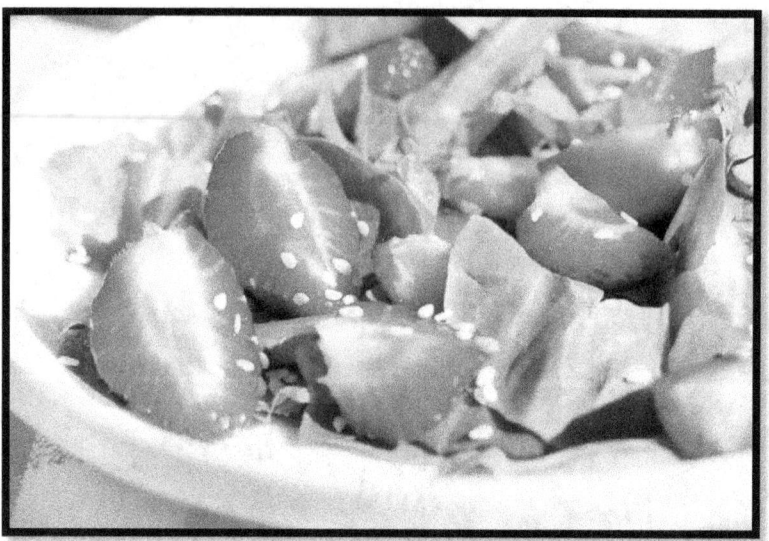

Ingredients:

- 5 cups fresh baby spinach, packed
- 2 green onions, sliced thin
- 1 ½ cups chopped fresh strawberries
- 1 tablespoon toasted sesame seeds
- 3 tablespoons olive oil
- 2 tablespoons balsamic vinegar
- 1 tablespoon minced yellow onion
- Pinch dry mustard powder
- Salt and pepper to taste

Instructions:

1. Toss together the spinach and green onion in a large salad bowl.
2. Top with the chopped strawberries and toasted sesame seeds.
3. Whisk together the remaining ingredients and drizzle over the salad just before serving.

Corn and Black Bean Salad

Servings: 6

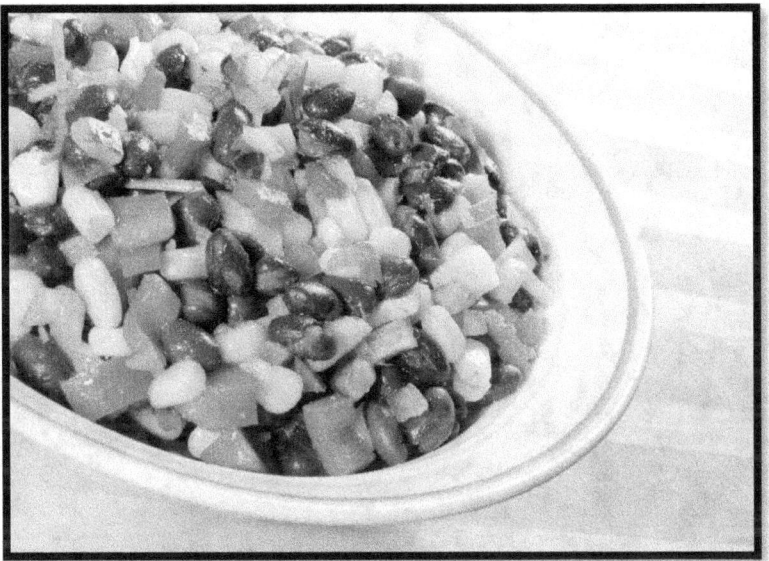

Ingredients:

- 2 (15 ounce) cans black beans, rinsed and drained
- 3 large ears of corn, cooked and kernels cut off
- 2 medium red bell peppers, cored and diced
- 2 tablespoons diced red onion
- 1 teaspoon minced garlic
- ½ cup extra-virgin olive oil
- 1/3 cup fresh lime juice
- 1 teaspoon fresh lime zest
- ½ cup fresh chopped cilantro
- Salt and pepper to taste

Instructions:

1. Combine the beans, corn, red pepper, garlic and onion in a mixing bowl.
2. Toss with the salt, pepper, olive oil, lime juice, lime zest and cilantro.
3. Cover and chill for several hours before serving.

Coconut Vegetable Curry

Servings: 4

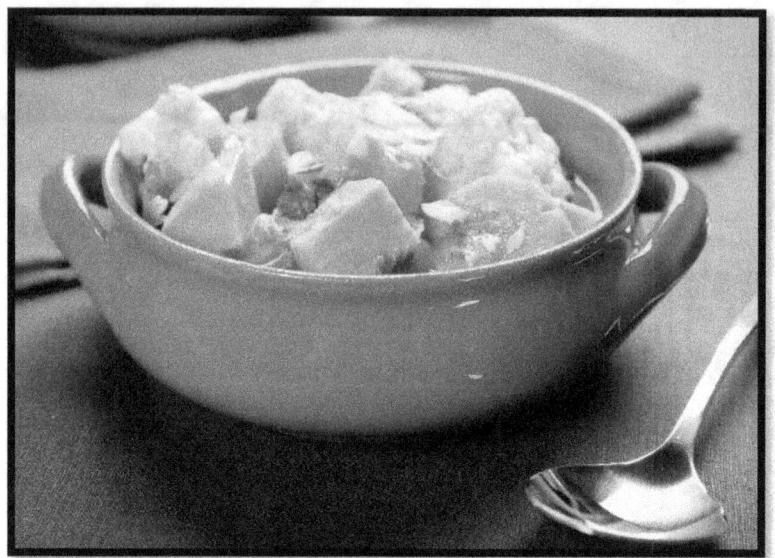

Ingredients:

- 1 tablespoon olive oil
- 1 medium yellow onion, chopped
- ½ cup chopped carrots
- 1 cup chopped cauliflower florets
- 1 tablespoon fresh grated ginger
- 1 tablespoon minced garlic
- Salt and pepper to taste
- 1 tablespoon curry powder
- 1 cup vegetable broth
- 2 (14.5 ounce) cans light coconut milk
- ½ cup diced tomato

Instructions:

1. Heat the oil in a large saucepan over medium heat.
2. Add the onion, carrot, cauliflower, ginger and garlic. Cook for 5 to 6 minutes until tender.
3. Season with salt and pepper to taste then stir in the curry powder, vegetable broth and coconut milk.

4. Simmer over medium-low heat for 12 to 15 minutes until the vegetables are tender.
5. Stir in the tomatoes and adjust seasonings to taste. Serve hot over steamed brown rice.

Apple Pecan Chicken Salad

Servings: 4

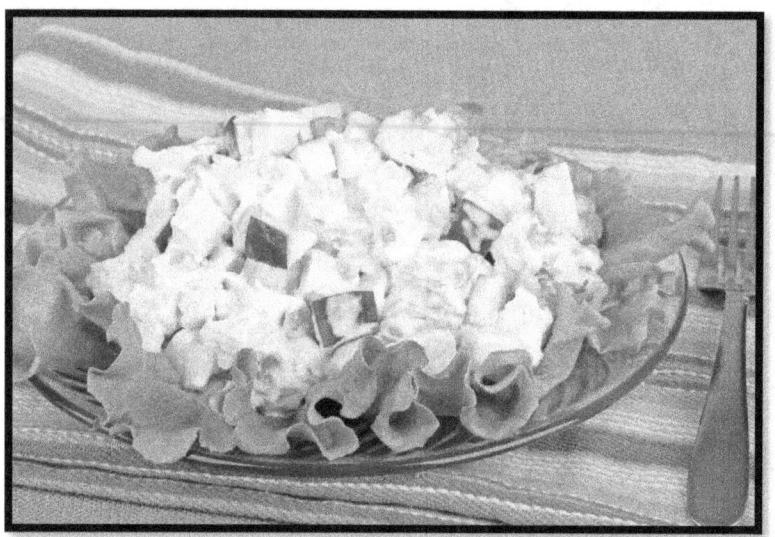

Ingredients:

- 1 lbs. boneless skinless chicken breast, cooked and chopped
- ½ cup diced red onion
- 1 small red apple, cored and diced
- ¼ cup diced celery
- ¼ cup finely chopped pecans
- ½ cup plain Greek yogurt
- 1 tablespoon fresh lemon juice
- ¼ teaspoon garlic powder
- Salt and pepper to taste

Instructions:

1. Toss together the chicken, red onion, apple, celery and pecans in a mixing bowl.
2. In a separate bowl, whisk together the remaining ingredients then toss with the chicken mixture.
3. Cover and chill for 1 hour then serve over a bed of lettuce.

Hearty Beef and Veggie Stew

Servings: 8 to 10

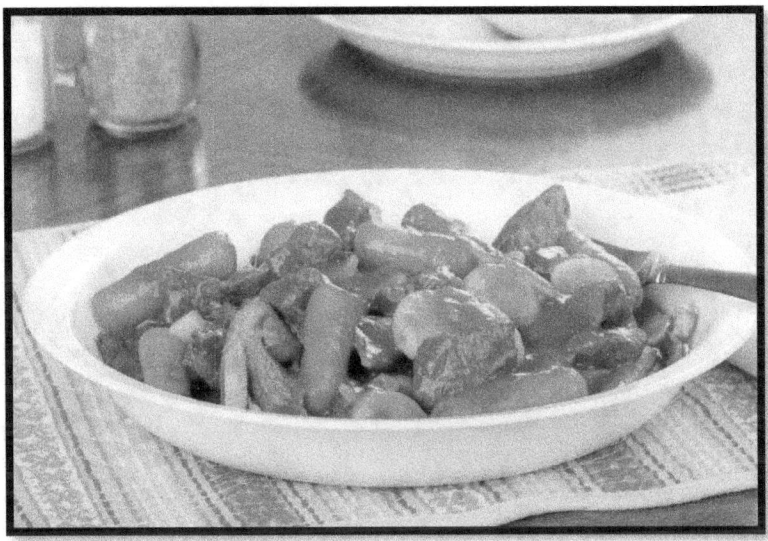

Ingredients:

- 2 tablespoons olive oil
- 4 lbs. beef stew meat, chopped
- Salt and pepper to taste
- 2 tablespoons whole wheat flour
- 4 cups beef broth
- 2 sprigs fresh thyme
- 3 bay leaves
- 2 large yellow onions, chopped
- 3 large carrots, peeled and sliced
- 1 tablespoon minced garlic

Instructions:

1. Preheat the oven to 350°F.
2. Heat the oil in a large Dutch oven over high heat.
3. Season the beef with salt and pepper to taste then place it in the hot Dutch oven.
4. Cook for 2 to 3 minutes on each side, turning often, until evenly browned – about 8 to 10 minutes total.
5. Stir in the flour to coat the meat then add the beef broth, thyme, and bay leaf.

6. Bring to a boil then stir in the onion, carrot and garlic.
7. Cover and transfer to the oven – cook for 1 ½ hours until the beef is tender.

Avocado Mango Spring Salad

Servings: 4

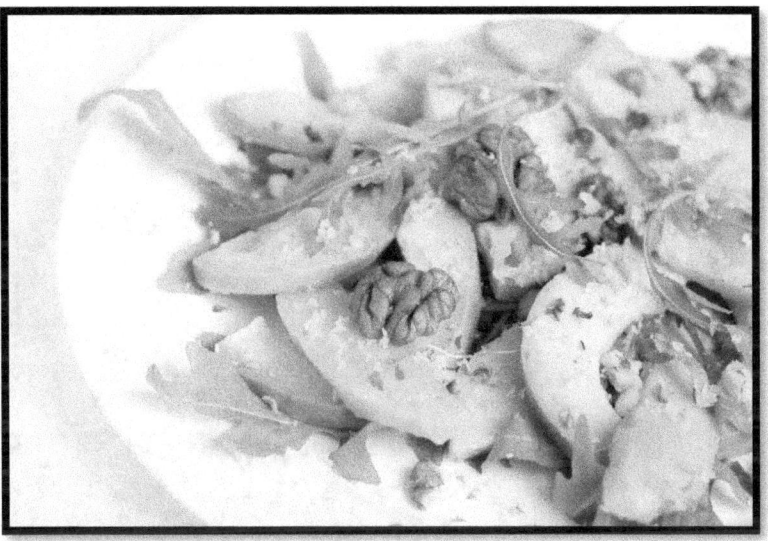

Ingredients:

- 5 cups fresh spring greens, packed
- ½ ripe mango, pitted and sliced thin
- ½ ripe avocado, pitted and sliced thin
- 1/3 cup toasted walnut halves, coarsely chopped
- 3 tablespoons extra-virgin olive oil
- 2 tablespoons red wine vinegar
- 1 teaspoon lemon juice
- 1 teaspoon honey
- Salt and pepper to taste

Instructions:

1. Divide the spring greens among plates and top with slices of mango and avocado.
2. Sprinkle the walnuts over the salads.
3. Whisk together the remaining ingredients and drizzle over the salads to serve.

Chilled Tomato Gazpacho

Servings: 6

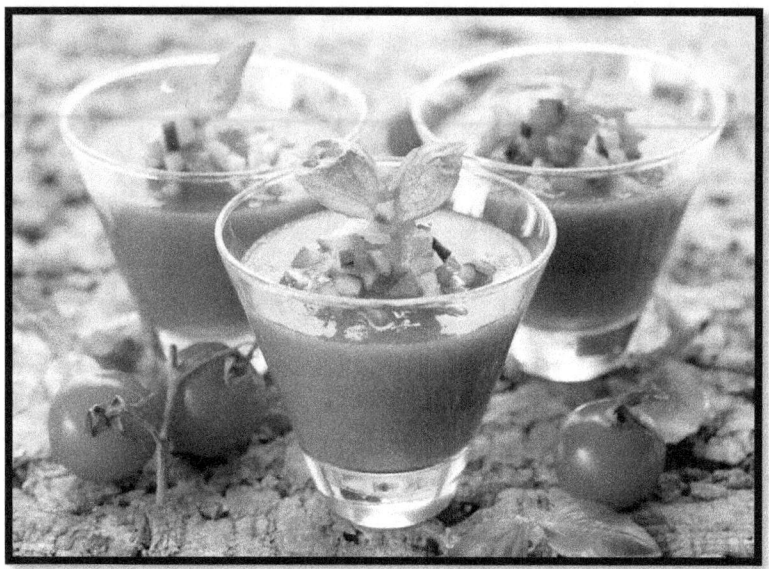

Ingredients:

- 2 lbs. ripe tomatoes, halved
- 1 medium seedless cucumber, peeled and diced
- 1 red bell pepper, cored and diced
- 1 cup diced red onion
- 1 cup cold water
- ¼ cup extra-virgin olive oil
- ¼ cup Sherry wine vinegar
- 1 teaspoon minced garlic
- ½ teaspoon ground cumin

Instructions:

1. Cover a bowl with a mesh strainer and squeeze the tomato halves into the strainer.
2. Use a wooden spoon to press on the tomato solids, straining the juice into the bowl – you should have about ½ cup.
3. Discard the tomato seeds and chop the flesh.
4. Combine the tomato juice and chopped tomato on a bowl and stir in the remaining ingredients.
5. Cover and let rest for 1 hour.

6. Transfer the mixture to a food processor, in batches if necessary, and pulse until finely chopped but not pureed.
7. Season with salt and pepper to taste and chill for several hours before serving.

Oven-Baked Rosemary Chicken

Servings: 6

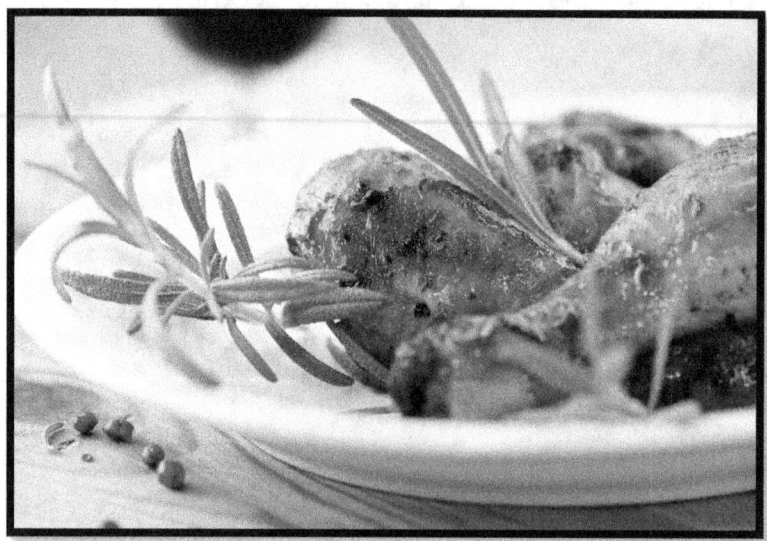

Ingredients:

- 3 lbs. chicken thighs and drumsticks
- 2 tablespoons olive oil
- 1 large yellow onion, chopped
- 1 cup sliced carrot
- 1 cup diced yellow potato
- 2 tablespoons dried rosemary
- ¼ cup chicken broth
- Salt and pepper to taste

Instructions:

1. Preheat the oven to 400°F.
2. Heat the oil in a large skillet over medium-high heat.
3. Season the chicken with salt and pepper to taste then place it in the skillet.
4. Cook the chicken for 2 to 3 minutes until browned then turn and brown on the other side.
5. Combine the vegetables in a rectangular glass baking dish and arrange the chicken on top.
6. Sprinkle with rosemary and drizzle with chicken broth.

7. Roast for 30 minutes then turn the chicken and roast for another 20 to 25 minutes until the juices run clear.

Balsamic-Grilled Salmon Steaks

Servings: 4

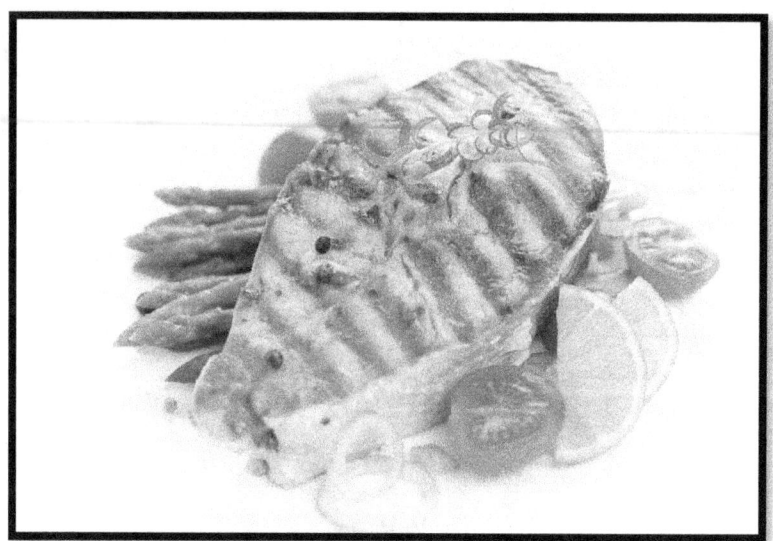

Ingredients:

- 2 tablespoons balsamic vinegar
- 2 tablespoons raw honey
- 1 tablespoon olive oil
- 1 teaspoon salt
- ¼ teaspoon black pepper
- 4 (6 ounce) salmon steaks, 1-inch thick

Instructions:

1. Combine the vinegar, honey, olive oil, salt and pepper in a plastic freezer bag.
2. Add the salmon steaks and turn to coat.
3. Chill the salmon steaks for 1 hour to marinate.
4. Preheat the grill to medium heat and brush the grates with olive oil.
5. Place the steaks on the grill and cook for 5 to 7 minutes on each side until the flesh flakes easily with a fork.

Baked Halibut with Mango Salsa

Servings: 4

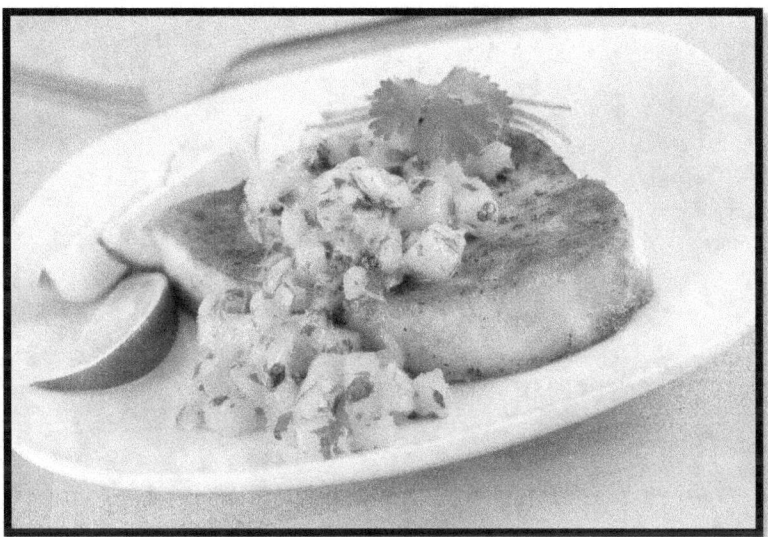

Ingredients:

- 4 (6 ounce) boneless halibut fillets
- 1 tablespoon olive oil
- Salt and pepper to taste
- ½ large lemon, sliced thin
- 1 large ripe mango, pitted and diced
- 3 tablespoons minced red onion
- 3 tablespoons fresh chopped cilantro
- 1 tablespoon fresh lemon juice

Instructions:

1. Preheat the oven to 350°F and line a baking sheet with parchment.
2. Rinse the fillets in cool water then pat dry with paper towel.
3. Brush the fillets with olive oil then season with salt and pepper to taste.
4. Place a slice of lemon on each fillet and bake for 12 to 15 minutes until the flesh flakes easily with a fork.
5. Combine the remaining ingredients in a bowl and serve over the cooked fish.

Broiled Lamb Chops

Servings: 4

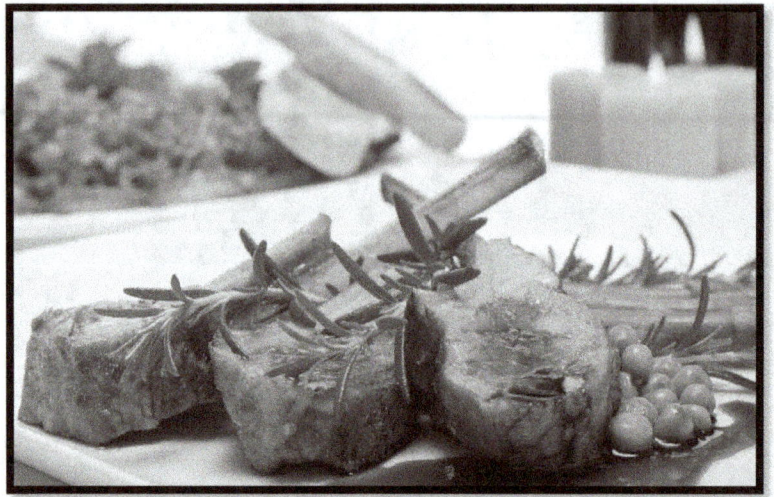

Ingredients:

- 1 ½ tablespoons minced garlic
- 3 tablespoons olive oil
- 2 teaspoon fresh chopped rosemary
- Salt and pepper to taste
- 12 lamb rib chops (2 to 2 ½ ounces each)

Instructions:

1. Preheat the broiler in your oven to high heat and place the oven rack in the highest position.
2. Combine the garlic, olive oil, and rosemary in a food processor and pulse to chop.
3. Season the lamb chops with salt and pepper to taste then coat in the garlic mixture.
4. Place the chops on a baking sheet and broil for 3 minutes per side for medium-rare.

Asian-Style Turkey Burgers

Servings: 4

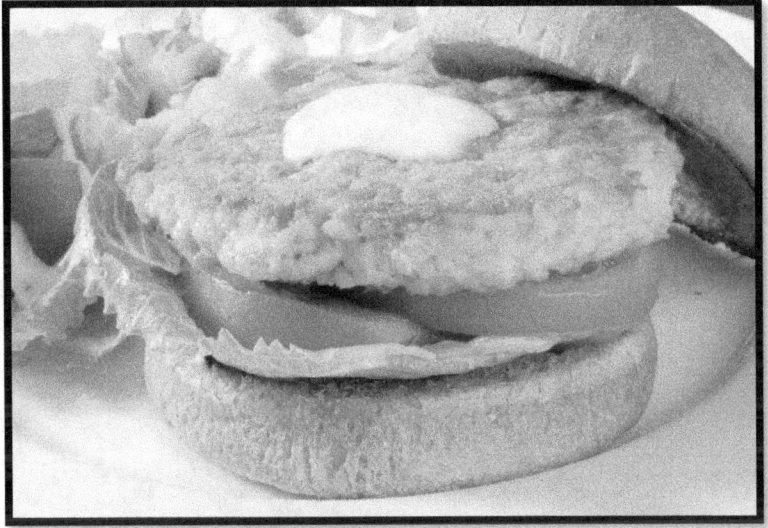

Ingredients:

- 12 ounces lean ground turkey
- ¼ cup whole-wheat breadcrumbs
- 2 tablespoons hoisin sauce
- 2 green onions, sliced thin
- 1 tablespoon fresh grated ginger
- 1 teaspoon minced ginger
- ¼ teaspoon salt
- ¼ cup plain Greek yogurt
- ¾ teaspoon low-sodium soy sauce
- ¼ teaspoon sesame oil

Instructions:

1. Preheat the broiler in your oven to high heat.
2. Combine the turkey, breadcrumbs, hoisin, green onions, ginger, garlic and salt in a mixing bowl.
3. Stir well then shape into ½-inch thick patties by hand.
4. Broil the turkey burgers for 4 to 6 minutes on each side until cooked through.
5. Whisk together the yogurt, soy sauce and sesame oil in a small bowl.

6. Serve the burgers hot on whole-wheat hamburger buns with a dollop of the flavored yogurt blend.

Almond-Crusted Tilapia

Servings: 4

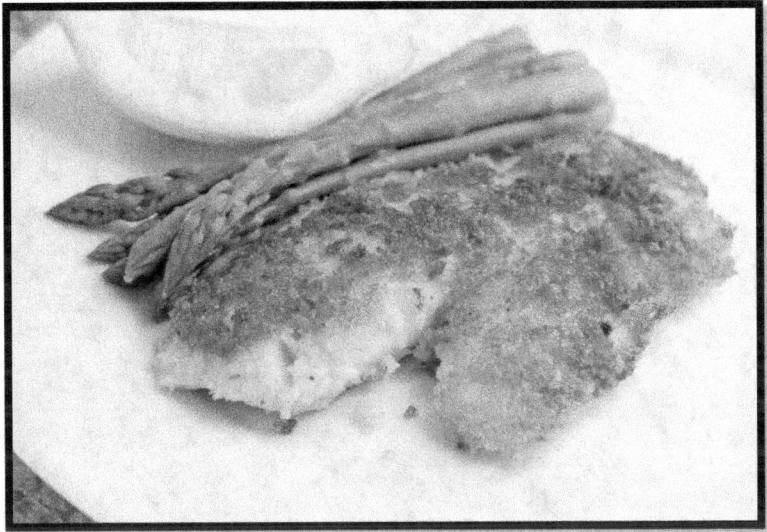

Ingredients:

- 4 (6 ounce) boneless tilapia fillets
- ¼ cup almond flour
- 3 tablespoons finely chopped almonds
- ½ teaspoon salt
- ¼ teaspoon freshly ground pepper
- 1 large egg, whisked

Instructions:

1. Preheat the oven to 350°F and line a baking sheet with parchment.
2. Rinse the fillets in cool water then pat dry with paper towel.
3. Stir together the almond flour, almonds, salt and pepper in a shallow dish.
4. Whisk the egg in a shallow dish then dip the fillets in egg.
5. Dredge the fillets in the almond flour mixture then place them on the baking sheet.
6. Bake for 12 to 15 minutes until the flesh flakes easily with a fork.

Ginger Beef and Veggie Stir-Fry

Servings: 4

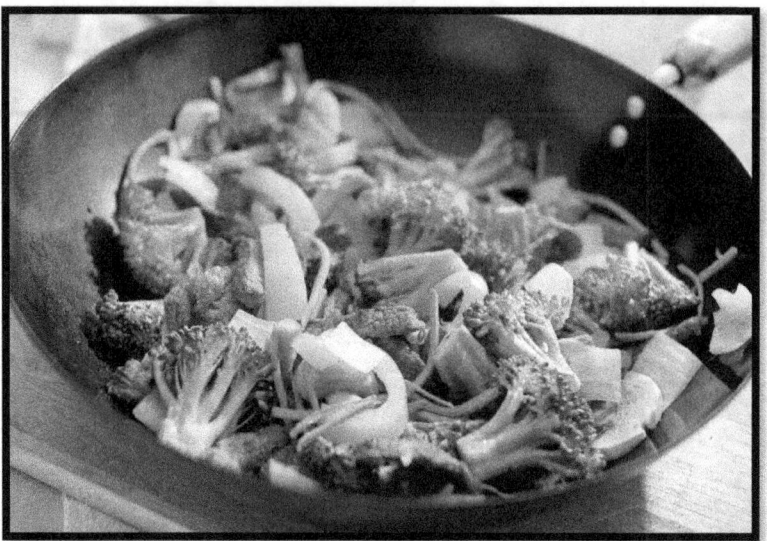

Ingredients:

- 1 lbs. sirloin beef, sliced ¼-inch thick
- 2 teaspoons cornstarch
- 4 tablespoons olive oil, divided
- 3 cups chopped broccoli florets
- 1 small yellow onion, chopped
- 1 small yellow pepper, cored and chopped
- 1 tablespoon minced ginger
- 1 tablespoon minced garlic
- ½ cup beef broth
- 1 tablespoon fish sauce
- 1 teaspoon honey

Instructions:

1. Place the beef in a plastic freezer bag and toss with the cornstarch until coated.
2. Heat 2 tablespoons of oil in a large skillet or wok over high heat.
3. Add the broccoli and sauté for 6 to 7 minutes until crisp-tender then spoon into a bowl.
4. Reheat the skillet with another tablespoon of oil.

5. Add the onions and yellow pepper and cook for 4 to 5 minutes until the onions are translucent.
6. Transfer the vegetables to the bowl with the broccoli.
7. Add the remaining tablespoon of oil along with the ginger and garlic.
8. Cook for 1 minute then arrange the beef in the skillet in a single layer.
9. Cook for 1 ½ minutes until browned then flip the slices and cook for another 30 to 60 seconds.
10. Remove the beef to the bowl with the vegetables.
11. Whisk together the remaining ingredients and pour into the skillet.
12. Heat for 2 minutes until thick and bubbling then toss in the beef and vegetables.
13. Cook for 1 to 2 minutes until heated through then serve with steamed brown rice.

Curried Lentil Stew

Servings: 6

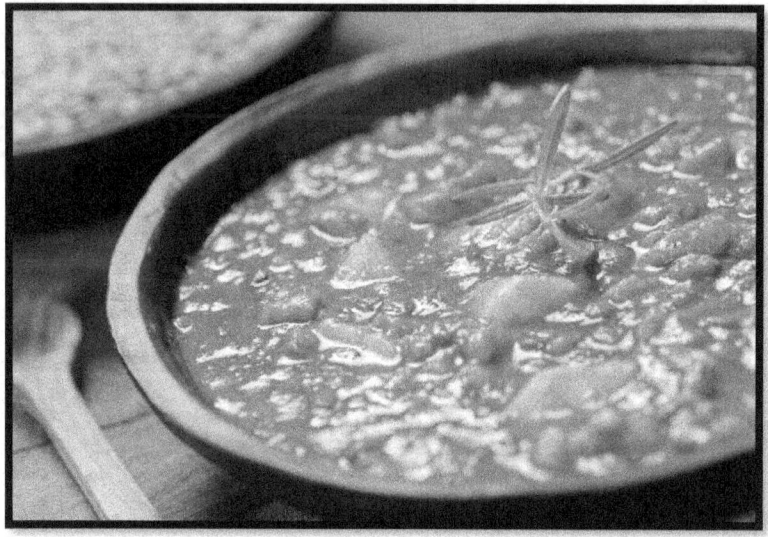

Ingredients:

- 1 tablespoon olive oil
- 1 large yellow onion, chopped
- 1 medium carrot, peeled and diced
- 2 teaspoons minced garlic
- 2 ½ tablespoons curry powder
- 1 cup red lentils (rinsed well)
- 4 ¼ cups water, divided
- 1 (15 ounce) can chickpeas, rinsed and drained
- 2 teaspoons lemon juice
- 2 tablespoons coconut oil
- Salt and pepper to taste

Instructions:

1. Heat the oil in a heavy skillet over medium heat.
2. Add the carrot and onion and cook for 4 to 5 minutes until the onion is translucent.
3. Stir in the garlic and cook for another 2 to 3 minutes.
4. Add the curry powder and cook for 1 minute then stir in the lentils and 4 cups water.
5. Season with salt and pepper to taste then bring to a boil.

6. Reduce heat and simmer for 30 minutes until the lentils are tender.
7. Combine the chickpeas, lemon juice, coconut oil, and remaining ¼ cup water in a food processor.
8. Blend smooth then stir into the skillet and adjust seasonings to taste. Serve hot.

Chapter Four: 30-Day Meal Plan

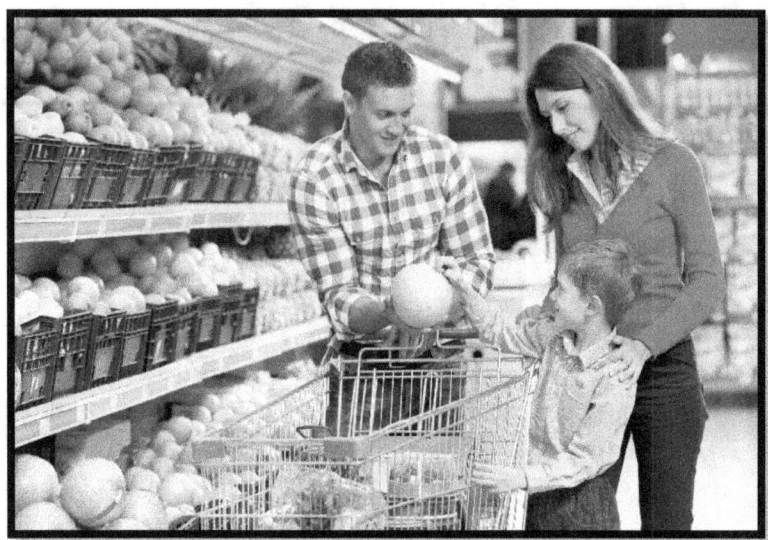

Making changes to your diet can be a challenge, especially if you are used to a certain routine. It is important to understand, however, that you will not get better unless you remove certain foods from your diet and replace them with other healthier foods. The recipes from the previous chapter are just a few examples of the many meal options you are still able to enjoy without exacerbating your condition. In fact, incorporating recipes like these into your everyday diet will help to improve your symptom or even reverse your condition entirely. If you need a little help getting started with a diabetic diet, use the 30-day meal plan provided in this chapter. Feel free to swap out the recipes listed for others in this book as you see fit.

30-Day Meal Plan to Reverse Diabetes			
Week 1	**Breakfast**	**Lunch**	**Dinner**
Day 1	Whole Wheat Toast with Jelly	Tuna Salad on Lettuce	Balsamic-Grilled Salmon Steaks
Day 2	Tropical Fruit Smoothie	Chilled Tomato Gazpacho	Chicken Burger with Side Salad
Day 3	Gluten-Free Banana Bread	Avocado Mango Spring Salad	Broiled Lamb Chops

Day 4	Vegetable Egg White Omelet	Hearty Beef and Veggie Stew	Almond-Crusted Tilapia
Day 5	Almond Flour Blueberry Muffins	Veggie and Hummus Pita Pocket	Salad with Grilled Chicken
Day 6	Tomato Basil Omelet	Apple Pecan Chicken Salad	Baked Halibut with Mango Salsa
Day 7	Steel Cut Oats with Sliced Banana	Coconut Vegetable Curry	Oven-Baked Rosemary Chicken
Week 2	**Breakfast**	**Lunch**	**Dinner**
Day 1	Mixed Vegetable Frittata	Low-Sodium Canned Soup	Asian-Style Turkey Burgers
Day 2	Blueberry Yogurt Parfait	Spinach Salad with Strawberries	Grilled Fish and Steamed Veggies
Day 3	Coconut Flour Banana Pancakes	Greek Salad with Chicken	Ginger Beef and Veggie Stir-Fry
Day 4	Scrambled Eggs with Chopped Veggies	Cream of Broccoli Soup	Curried Lentil Stew
Day 5	Raspberry Coconut Smoothie	Corn and Black Bean Salad	Broiled Steak with Side Salad
Day 6	Vegetable Egg White Omelet	Turkey Burger on Whole-Wheat Bun	Oven-Baked Rosemary Chicken
Day 7	Baked Broccoli Egg Cups	Chilled Tomato Gazpacho	Whole-Grain Pasta with Tomato Sauce
Week 3	**Breakfast**	**Lunch**	**Dinner**
Day 1	Fresh Fruit	Tossed Salad with Fruit and Nuts	Balsamic-Grilled Salmon Steaks
Day 2	Almond Flour Blueberry Muffins	Hearty Beef and Veggie Stew	Grass-Fed Beef Burger with Veggies
Day 3	Steel Cut Oats with Sliced Banana	Avocado Mango Spring Salad	Broiled Lamb Chops
Day 4	Tropical Fruit Smoothie	Tuna Salad on Lettuce	Baked Halibut with Mango Salsa
Day 5	Mixed Vegetable Frittata	Coconut Vegetable Curry	Salad with Grilled Chicken
Day 6	Whole Wheat Toast with Jelly	Greek Salad with Chicken	Grilled Shrimp with Vegetables
Day 7	Coconut Flour Banana Pancakes	Corn and Black Bean Salad	Asian-Style Turkey Burgers

Week 4	Breakfast	Lunch	Dinner
Day 1	Blueberry Yogurt Parfait	Apple Pecan Chicken Salad	Chicken Burger with Side Salad
Day 2	Gluten-Free Banana Bread	Low-Sodium Canned Soup	Almond-Crusted Tilapia
Day 3	Whole-Grain Cereal with Almond Milk	Spinach Salad with Strawberries	Whole-Grain Pasta with Pesto
Day 4	Baked Broccoli Egg Cups	Hearty Beef and Veggie Stew	Curried Lentil Stew
Day 5	Scrambled Eggs with Chopped Veggies	Veggie and Hummus Pita Pocket	Broiled Steak with Side Salad
Day 6	Raspberry Coconut Smoothie	Cream of Broccoli Soup	Grilled Chicken Tacos
Day 7	Tomato Basil Omelet	Avocado Mango Spring Salad	Ginger Beef and Veggie Stir-Fry

Conclusion

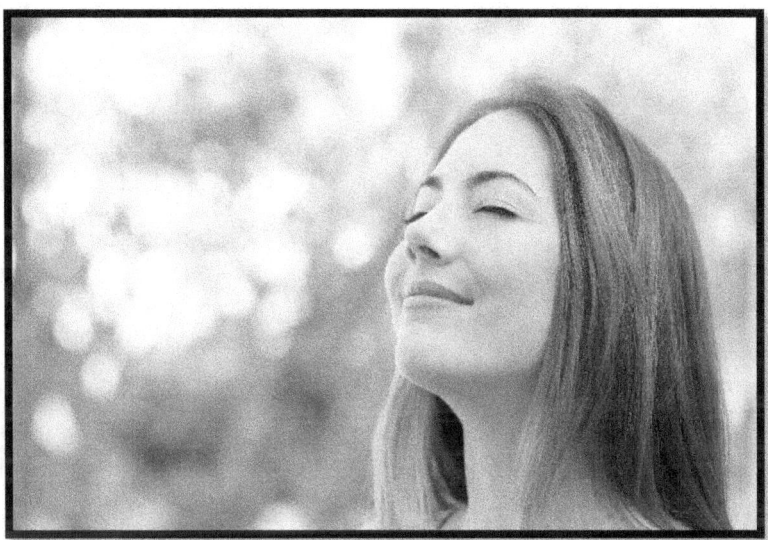

After reading this book you should have a basic understanding of the differences between the three types of diabetes as well as their causes. Additionally, you should see and understand how making simple changes to your diet and lifestyle can have a positive effect on Type II diabetes, perhaps going so far as to reverse the condition entirely. In following the tips in this book and utilizing the recipes provided, you have the tools and knowledge you need to reverse your Type II diabetes in as little as 30 days. If you are ready to take control of your life and to improve your health, don't wait any longer – get started today using the 30-day meal plan provided in Chapter Four. Good luck!